48 Juice Recipes to Correct Vision Problems:

Natures Solution to the Loss of Vision and Eye Sight Problems

By

Joe Correa CSN

COPYRIGHT

This publication is designed to provide accurate and authoritative information in regard to the subject matter covered. It is sold with the understanding that neither the author nor the publisher is engaged in rendering medical advice. If medical advice or assistance is needed, consult with a doctor. This book is considered a guide and should not be used in any way detrimental to your health. Consult with a physician before starting this nutritional plan to make sure it's right for you.

ACKNOWLEDGEMENTS

This book is dedicated to my friends and family that have had mild or serious illnesses so that you may find a solution and make the necessary changes in your life.

48 Juice Recipes to Correct Vision Problems:

Natures Solution to the Loss of Vision and Eye Sight Problems

By

Joe Correa CSN

CONTENTS

Copyright

Acknowledgements

About The Author

Introduction

48 Juice Recipes to Correct Vision Problems: Natures Solution to the Loss of Vision and Eye Sight Problems

Additional Titles from This Author

ABOUT THE AUTHOR

After years of Research, I honestly believe in the positive effects that proper nutrition can have over the body and mind. My knowledge and experience has helped me live healthier throughout the years and which I have shared with family and friends. The more you know about eating and drinking healthier, the sooner you will want to change your life and eating habits.

Nutrition is a key part in the process of being healthy and living longer so get started today. The first step is the most important and the most significant.

INTRODUCTION

48 Juice Recipes to Correct Vision Problems: Natures Solution to the Loss of Vision and Eye Sight Problems

By Joe Correa CSN

While degraded vision is something that most of us eventually have to deal with as we age, the causes of more severe vision loss vary. Some studies show that when you are over the age of 65 you will be 25 percent more likely to experience some form of vision loss.

The main causes of vision loss are:

- Macular Degradation in one or both eyes, mainly due to age;
- Cataracts, which cause blurry vision or double vision. This is more common with aging and can and should be surgically removed when it causes problems;
- Diabetic Retinopathy, which is a severe complication, associated with diabetes;
- Side effects of a stroke

While some off the causes mentioned above can be treated with surgery there are other remedies for age related and regular vision impairment that can be aided with certain eye exercises as well as certain superfoods.

Some foods have shown to be more effective than others at aiding vision improvement.

I have used those foods to come up with tasty juice recipes that you can make by yourself at home. The recipes in this book offer a magnificent variety of both flavor and natural goodness, which should aid your efforts to improve the function of your eyes.

This book is a collection of recipes that incorporate vitamins and minerals directly from Mother Nature. Zesty oranges, beneficial leafy greens, carrots, and other fruits and vegetables in various combinations will satisfy every taste. Get started and enjoy!

48 JUICE RECIPES TO CORRECT VISION PROBLEMS

1.   Fennel Spinach Juice

Ingredients:

1 cup of fennel, chopped

1 cup of collard greens, torn

3 large green apples, cored

1 cup of fresh spinach, torn

Preparation:

Wash the fennel bulb and trim off the wilted outer layers. Cut into small chunks and fill the measuring cup. Reserve the rest in the refrigerator.

In a large colander, combine collard greens and spinach. Rinse thoroughly under cold running water and drain. Torn with hands and set aside.

Wash the apples and cut in half. Remove the core and cut into bite-sized pieces. Set aside.

Now, combine fennel, collard greens, spinach and apple in a juicer. Process until well juiced.

Transfer to a serving glass and refrigerate for 15 minutes before serving.

Enjoy!

Nutritional information per serving: Kcal: 220, Protein: 5g, Carbs: 66.3g, Fats: 1.3g

2.   Cucumber Broccoli Juice

Ingredients:

1 cup of cucumber, sliced

2 cups of broccoli, chopped

1 cup of Brussels sprouts

1 teaspoon of olive oil

Preparation:

Wash the cucumber and cut into thin slices. Fill the measuring cup and reserve the rest for later. Set aside.

Wash the broccoli and trim off the outer layers. Cut into small pieces and set aside.

Wash the Brussels sprouts and trim off the outer wilted leaves. Cut in half and set aside.

Now, combine Cucumber, Broccoli and Brussels sprouts in a juicer and process until well juiced and add one teaspoon of olive oil before serving.

Serve immediately.

Enjoy!

Nutrition information per serving: Kcal: 74, Protein: 8.4g, Carbs: 21.8g, Fats: 1g

3. Cauliflower Broccoli Juice

Ingredients:

1 cup of cauliflower, chopped

1 cup of fresh basil, torn

2 cups of broccoli, chopped

1 medium-sized red apple, cored

1 large lemon, peeled

Preparation:

Trim off the outer leaves of a cauliflower. Wash it and fill and cut into small pieces. Fill the measuring cup and reserve the rest in the refrigerator.

Wash the broccoli and chop into small pieces. Set aside.

Wash the apple and cut lengthwise in half. Remove the core and cut into bite-sized pieces. Set aside.

Peel the lemon and cut lengthwise in half. Set aside.

Now, combine cauliflower, basil, broccoli, apple and lemon in a juicer. Process until well juiced and transfer to a serving glass.

Add few ice cubes and serve immediately.

Enjoy!

Nutritional information per serving: Kcal: 156, Protein: 9g, Carbs: 46.4g, Fats: 1.5g

4.   Zucchini Basil Juice

Ingredients:

1 small zucchini, chopped

1 cup of mustard greens, chopped

2 cups of fresh basil, chopped

1 whole lime, peeled

1 whole cucumber, sliced

Preparation:

Peel the zucchini and cut into bite-sized pieces. Set aside.

Combine fresh basil and mustard greens in a large colander. Wash thoroughly under cold running water. Roughly chop it and soak in lukewarm water for 10 minutes.

Peel the lime and cut lengthwise in half. Set aside.

Wash the cucumber and cut into thin slices. Set aside.

Now, combine zucchini, basil, mustard greens, lime, and cucumber in a juicer and process until well juiced. Transfer to a serving glass and refrigerate for 10 minutes before serving.

Enjoy!

Nutritional information per serving: Kcal: 126, Protein: 7.5g, Carbs: 38.8g, Fats: 1.4g

5.   Cauliflower Avocado Juice

Ingredients:

5 cauliflower flowerets, chopped

1 cup of avocado, cubed

1 whole lime, peeled

1 whole leek, chopped

Preparation:

Wash the cauliflower flowerets thoroughly and chop into small pieces. Set aside.

Peel the avocado and cut in half. Remove the pit and cut into small cubes. Fill the measuring cup and reserve the rest in the refrigerator. Set aside.

Peel the lime and cut lengthwise in half. Set aside.

Wash the leek and cut into small pieces. Set aside.

Now, combine cauliflower, avocado, lime, and leek in a juicer and process until juiced. Transfer to a serving glass and refrigerate for 10 minutes before serving.

Enjoy!

Nutritional information per serving: Kcal: 268, Protein: 5.7g, Carbs: 32.4g, Fats: 22.5g

6.   Apple Kale Juice

Ingredients:

1 medium-sized red apple, cored

1 cup of cucumber, sliced

2 cups of fresh kale, chopped

1 cup of watercress, torn

1 cup of fresh parsley, torn

1 oz of water

Preparation:

Wash the cucumber and cut into thin slices. Fill the measuring cup and reserve the rest for later. Set aside.

Wash the apple and cut lengthwise in half. Remove the core and cut into bite-sized pieces. Set aside.

Wash the kale thoroughly under cold running water. Chop into small pieces and set aside.

Combine watercress and parsley in a colander. Rinse well under cold running water and torn with hands. Set aside.

Now, combine cucumber, apple, kale, watercress, and parsley in a juicer and process until juiced. Transfer to a serving glass and stir in the water. Add some ice before serving.

Enjoy!

Nutritional information per serving: Kcal: 150, Protein: 9.1g, Carbs: 40.8g, Fats: 2g

7.   Carrots Orange Juice

Ingredients:

2 medium-sized carrots, sliced

2 cups of broccoli, chopped

1 large orange, peeled

1 whole lemon, peeled

1 small ginger knob, peeled

Preparation:

Wash and peel the carrot. Cut into thin slices and set aside.

Trim off the outer leaves of the broccoli. Wash it and cut into bite-sized pieces. Set aside.

Peel the orange and divide into wedges. Cut each wedge in half and set aside.

Peel the lemon and cut lengthwise in half. Set aside.

Peel the ginger knob and set aside.

Now, combine carrots, broccoli, orange, lemon, and, ginger knob in a juicer. Process until juiced.

Transfer to a serving glass and refrigerate for 15 minutes before serving.

Nutritional information per serving: Kcal: 162, Protein: 8.7g, Carbs: 51.8g, Fats: 1.4g

8.　Kale Broccoli Juice

Ingredients:

1 cup of kale, roughly chopped

2 cups of broccoli, chopped

1 small green apple, cored

1 medium-sized asparagus spears, trimmed

1 whole lemon, peeled

1 cup of fresh parsley, torn

Preparation:

Rinse the kale under cold running water. Slightly drain and torn with hands. Set aside.

Trim off the outer leaves of the broccoli. Wash it and cut into bite-sized pieces. Set aside.

Wash the apple and cut in half. Remove the core and cut into bite-sized pieces. Set aside.

Wash the asparagus and trim off the woody ends. Cut into small pieces and set aside.

Peel the lemon and cut lengthwise in half. Set aside.

Add parsley in a colander. Rinse well under cold running water and torn with hands. Set aside.

Now, combine kale, broccoli, apple, asparagus, lemon and parsley in a juicer. Process until juiced.

Transfer to a serving glass and refrigerate for 15 minutes before serving.

Nutritional information per serving: Kcal: 154, Protein: 11.1g, Carbs: 45.3g, Fats: 2.1g

9.   Zucchini Parsnip Juice

Ingredients:

1 cup of cucumber, sliced

1 small zucchini, chopped

1 cup of parsnip, sliced

1 medium-sized carrot, sliced

¼ tsp of ginger, ground

Preparation:

Wash the cucumber and cut into slices. Fill the measuring cup and reserve the rest for later.

Peel the zucchini and cut into bite-sized pieces. Set aside.

Wash and slightly peel the parsnip. Cut into thin slices and fill the measuring cup. Reserve the rest for later. Set aside.

Wash and peel the carrot. Cut into thin slices and set aside.

Now, combine cucumber, zucchini, parsnip and carrot in a juicer and process until juiced.

Transfer to a serving glass and stir in the ginger. Refrigerate for 10 minutes before serving.

Enjoy!

Nutritional information per serving: Kcal: 161, Protein: 7g, Carbs: 48.1g, Fats 1.8g

10.   Carrot Apple Juice

Ingredients:

2 large carrots, sliced

2 small green apples, cored

1 small zucchini, chopped

1 large lime, peeled

¼ tsp of ginger, ground

Preparation:

Wash and peel the carrots. Cut into thin slices and set aside.

Wash the apple and cut in half. Remove the core and cut into bite-sized pieces. Set aside.

Peel the zucchini and cut into thin slices. Set aside.

Peel the lime and cut lengthwise in half. Set aside.

Now, combine carrots, apples, zucchini and lime in a juicer. Process until well juiced. Transfer to a serving glass and stir in the ginger.

Enjoy!

Nutritional information per serving: Kcal: 161, Protein: 7g, Carbs: 48.1g, Fats: 1.8g

11.   Raspberries Basil Juice

Ingredients:

2 medium-sized carrots, sliced

2 cups of raspberries

1 cup of fresh basil, torn

1 whole lemon, peeled

1 small Granny Smith's apple, cored

Preparation:

Wash and peel the carrots. Cut into thin slices and set aside.

Using a colander, rinse the raspberries under cold running water. Slightly drain and set aside.

Wash the basil thoroughly and torn with hands. Set aside.

Peel the lemon and cut lengthwise in half. Set aside.

Wash the apple and cut in half. Remove the core and cut into bite-sized pieces. Set aside.

Now, combine carrots, raspberries, basil, lemon and apple in a juicer and process until juiced.

Transfer to a serving glass and add few ice cubes.

Serve immediately.

Enjoy!

Nutritional information per serving: Kcal: 223, Protein: 7.3g, Carbs: 79.5g, Fats: 2.8g

12.   Raspberry Carrot Juice

Ingredients:

1 cup of raspberries

1 cup of blackberries

1 cup of blueberries

2 large carrots, peeled and chopped

1 large orange, wedged

1 tsp of fresh rosemary, finely chopped

Preparation:

Using a colander, wash the raspberries in under cold running water. Slightly drain and set aside.

Combine blackberries and blueberries in a colander. Rinse under cold running water and drain. Set aside.

Wash the carrots and peel them. Cut into small chunks and set aside.

Peel the orange and divide into wedges. Set aside.

Now, combine raspberries, blueberries, blackberries, carrots, orange and rosemary in a juicer and process until well juiced. Transfer to a serving glass.

Refrigerate for 10 minutes before serving.

Nutritional information per serving: Kcal: 246, Protein: 7.6g, Carbs: 85.4g, Fats: 2.5g

13.   Collard greens Carrot Juice

Ingredients:

2 cup of cucumber, sliced

2 cups of collard greens, torn

1 cup of fresh parsley, chopped

3 medium-sized carrots, sliced

1 tsp of fresh rosemary, finely chopped

Preparation:

Wash the cucumber and cut into thin slices. Fill the measuring cup and reserve the rest for later. Set aside.

Wash the collard greens thoroughly under cold running water. Place them in a bowl and add 2 cups of boiling water. Let it soak for 10 minutes. Slightly drain and set aside.

Rinse the parsley under cold running water and chop into small pieces.

Wash and peel the carrot. Cut into thin slices and set aside.

Now, combine cucumber, collard greens, parsley, carrots, and rosemary in a juicer and process until juiced.

Transfer to a serving glass and refrigerate for 10 minutes before serving.

Nutritional information per serving: Kcal: 94, Protein: 6.3g, Carbs: 29g, Fats: 1.4g

14.   Avocado Collard Greens Juice

Ingredients

1 cup of avocado, cubed

2 cups of collard greens, torn

1 small Granny Smith's apple, cored

1 cup of watercress, torn

1 tsp of fresh rosemary, finely chopped

Preparation:

Peel the avocado and cut in half. Remove the pit and cut into small cubes. Fill the measuring cup and reserve the rest in the refrigerator. Set aside.

Wash the collard greens thoroughly under cold running water. Place them in a bowl and add 2 cups of boiling water. Let it soak for 10 minutes. Slightly drain and set aside.

Wash the apple and cut in half. Remove the core and cut into bite-sized pieces. Set aside.

Wash the watercress and torn with hands. Set aside.

Now, combine avocado, collard greens, apples, watercress

and rosemary in a juicer.

Process until well juiced and transfer to a serving glass. Refrigerate for 10 minutes before serving.

Nutritional information per serving: Kcal: 389, Protein: 8.1g, Carbs: 43.5g, Fats: 34.4g

15.   Mixed Berry Juice

Ingredients:

1 cup of cranberries

1 cup of blackberries

1 cup of blueberries

1 large lime, peeled

1 large cucumber, chopped

1 cup of parsnip, sliced

Preparation:

Combine cranberries, blackberries and blueberries in a colander. Rinse under cold running water and drain. Set aside.

Peel the lime and cut lengthwise in half. Set aside.

Wash the cucumber and cut into small chunks. Set aside.

Wash and slightly peel the parsnip. Cut into thin slices and fill the measuring cup. Reserve the rest for later. Set aside.

Now, combine cranberries, blackberries, blueberries, cucumber, lime and parsnip in a juicer and process until juiced. Transfer to serving glasses and stir in the water.

Add some ice or refrigerate for 15 minutes before serving.

Nutritional information per serving: Kcal: 243, Protein: 7g, Carbs: 82.3g, Fats: 2g

16.   Apple Cranberry Juice

Ingredients:

1 small Granny Smith's apple, chopped

1 cup of cranberries

1 cup of watercress, torn

½ cup of fresh spinach, torn

1 small ginger knob, peeled

Preparation:

Wash the apple and remove the core. Cut into bite-sized pieces and set aside.

Place the cranberries in a colander and rinse thoroughly. Slightly drain and set aside.

Wash watercress and spinach thoroughly under cold running water. Drain and torn with hands. Set aside.

Peel the ginger and set aside.

Now, combine apple, cranberries, watercress, spinach, and ginger in a juicer and process until well juiced. Transfer to a serving glass and stir in some water if you like. However, it is optional.

Refrigerate for 15 minutes before serving.

Enjoy!

Nutritional information per serving: Kcal: 249, Protein: 3.8g, Carbs: 86.1g, Fats: 0.9g

17. Fennel Collard Green Juice

Ingredients:

1 cup of fennel, chopped

1 cup of collard greens, torn

1 large green apple, cored

A handful of spinach

1 teaspoon of olive oil

Preparation:

Wash the fennel bulb and trim off the wilted outer layers. Cut into small chunks and fill the measuring cup. Reserve the rest in the refrigerator.

In a large colander, combine collard greens and spinach. Rinse thoroughly under cold running water and drain. Torn with hands and set aside.

Wash the apple and cut in half. Remove the core and cut into bite-sized pieces. Set aside.

Now, combine fennel, collard greens, spinach, and apple in a juicer. Process until well juiced.

Transfer to a serving glass and add one teaspoon of olive

oil and refrigerate for 15 minutes before serving.

Enjoy!

Nutritional information per serving: Kcal: 122, Protein: 3.9g, Carbs: 37.4g, Fats: 0.9g

18.   Avocado Kale Juice

Ingredients:

1 cup of fresh spinach, torn

1 cup of fresh kale, torn

1 cup of fresh parsley, torn

1 cup of cucumber, sliced

1 cup of avocado, chunked

¼ tsp of turmeric, ground

Preparation:

Combine spinach, kale, and parsley in a large colander. Rinse all under cold running water and slightly drain. Torn with hands and set aside.

Wash the cucumber and cut into thin slices. Set aside.

Peel the avocado and cut in half. Remove the pit and cut into small chunks. Fill the measuring cup and reserve the rest for later.

Now, combine spinach, kale, parsley, cucumber and avocado in a juicer and process until juiced. Transfer to a serving glass and stir in the turmeric.

Refrigerate for 10 minutes and serve.

Enjoy!

Nutritional information per serving: Kcal: 285, Protein: 17.3g, Carbs: 34.8g, Fats: 24.4g

19.   Grapefruit Carrots Juice

Ingredients:

1 cup of raspberries

2 large oranges, wedged

2 large carrots, peeled and chopped

1 whole grapefruit, wedged

1 small ginger knob

Preparation:

Using a colander rinse raspberries under cold running water and drain. Set aside.

Peel the orange and divide into wedges. Cut each wedge in half and set aside.

Wash the carrots and peel them. Cut into small chunks and set aside.

Peel the grapefruit and divide into wedges. Cut each wedge in half and set aside.

Now, combine raspberries, orange, carrots, grapefruit and ginger in a juicer and process until well juiced. Transfer to a serving glass and stir in the coconut water.

Enjoy!

Nutritional information per serving: Kcal: 304, Protein: 8.2g, Carbs: 99g, Fats: 1.9g

20.   Orange Celery Juice

Ingredients:

2 small oranges, wedged

2 medium-sized celery stalks

1 small apple, cored

1 cup of raspberries

1 small ginger knob

Preparation:

Peel the orange and divide into wedges. Set aside.

Wash the celery and cut into bite-sized pieces. Set aside.

Wash the apple and cut in half. Remove the core and cut into bite-sized pieces. Set aside.

Using a colander wash the raspberries in under cold running water. Slightly drain and set aside.

Now, combine orange, celery, apple, raspberries and ginger in a juicer and process until well juiced. Transfer to a serving glass and add some crushed ice.

Serve immediately.

Enjoy!

Nutrition information per serving: Kcal: 185, Protein: 4.5g, Carbs: 60.3g, Fats: 1.4g

21.   Romaine lettuce Spinach Juice

Ingredients:

1 cup of fresh coriander, chopped

1 cup of fresh spinach, torn

1 cup of Romaine lettuce, shredded

1 whole cucumber, sliced

1 teaspoon of olive oil

Preparation:

Combine coriander, spinach, and lettuce in a large colander. Wash thoroughly under cold running water and slightly drain. Roughly chop all and set aside.

Wash the cucumber and cut into thin slices. Set aside.

Now, combine coriander, spinach, lettuce, and cucumber in a juicer and process until well juiced.

Transfer to a serving glass and add one teaspoon of olive oil before serving.

Serve immediately.

Enjoy!

Nutrition information per serving: Kcal: 85, Protein: 10.3g, Carbs: 23.9g, Fats: 1.8g

22.   Carrot Cucumber Juice

Ingredients:

4 medium-sized carrots, sliced

1 whole lime, peeled

2 cups of cucumber, sliced

1 small zucchini, chopped

1 medium-sized orange, wedged

1 tbsp of honey

Preparation:

Wash and peel the carrots. Cut into thin slices and set aside.

Peel the lime and cut lengthwise in half. Set aside.

Wash the cucumber and cut into thin slices. Fill the measuring cup and reserve the rest for later.

Peel the zucchini and cut lengthwise in half. Scrape out the seeds and wash it. Cut into small pieces and set aside.

Peel the orange and divide into wedges. Cut each wedge in half and set aside.

Now, combine carrots, lime, cucumber, zucchini and orange in a juicer and process until juiced.

Transfer to a serving glass and stir in the honey.

Add some ice before serving.

Enjoy!

Nutrition information per serving: Kcal: 161, Protein: 5.8g, Carbs: 49.9g, Fats: 1.2g

23. Raspberries Oranges Juice

Ingredients:

4 large carrots, peeled and chopped

2 cups of raspberries

2 large oranges, wedged

¼ tsp of ginger, ground

Preparation:

Wash the carrots and peel them. Cut into small chunks and set aside.

Using a colander rinse the raspberries under cold running water and drain. Set aside.

Peel the oranges and divide into wedges. Set aside.

Now, combine carrots, raspberries and oranges in a juicer and process until well juiced. Transfer to a serving glass and stir in the ginger.

Refrigerate for 15 minutes before serving.

Enjoy!

Nutritional information per serving: Kcal: 274, Protein: 8.7g, Carbs: 96.3g, Fats: 2.6g

24.   Cauliflower Basil Juice

Ingredients:

2 cup of cauliflower, chopped

1 cup of fresh basil, torn

1 cup of beet greens, torn

1 cup of broccoli, chopped

1 large lemon, peeled

2 large oranges, wedged

1 medium-sized red apple, cored

Preparation:

Trim off the outer leaves of a cauliflower. Wash it and fill and cut into small pieces. Fill the measuring cup and reserve the rest in the refrigerator.

Combine basil and beet greens in a large colander. Rinse under cold running water and drain. Torn with hands and set aside.

Wash the broccoli and chop into small pieces. Set aside.

Peel the lemon and cut lengthwise in half. Set aside.

Peel the oranges and divide into wedges. Set aside.

Wash the apple and cut lengthwise in half. Remove the core and cut into bite-sized pieces. Set aside.

Now, combine cauliflower, basil, broccoli, beet greens, lemon, oranges and apple in a juicer. Process until well juiced and transfer to a serving glass.

Add few ice cubes and serve immediately.

Enjoy!

Nutritional information per serving: Kcal: 290, Protein: 13.1g, Carbs: 90.3g, Fats: 2g

25.   Apple Brussels sprouts Juice

Ingredients:

1 medium-sized apple, cored

1 cup of Brussels sprouts

1 medium-sized carrot, chopped

1 whole lemon, peeled

2 large oranges, wedged

2 oz of water

Preparation:

Wash the apple and cut lengthwise in half. Remove the core and cut into bite-sized pieces. Set aside.

Wash the Brussels sprouts and trim off the outer wilted leaves. Cut in half and set aside.

Wash and peel the carrot. Cut into small chunks and set aside.

Peel the lemon and cut lengthwise in half. Set aside.

Peel the orange and divide into wedges. Cut each wedge in half and set aside.

Now, combine apple, Brussels sprouts, carrot, lemon and oranges in a juicer. Process until nicely juiced. Transfer to a serving glass.

Add some ice or refrigerate for 10 minutes before serving.

Enjoy!

Nutritional information per serving: Kcal: 367, Protein: 11.6g, Carbs: 113.8g, Fats: 2g

26. Zucchini Broccoli Juice

Ingredients:

1 small zucchini, chopped

1 cup of broccoli, chopped

1 cup of Brussels sprouts

1 cup of cucumber, sliced

1 small ginger slice, peeled

1 teaspoon of olive oil

Preparation:

Wash the broccoli and trim off the outer layers. Cut into small pieces and set aside.

Peel the zucchini and cut into bite-sized pieces. Set aside.

Wash the Brussels sprouts and trim off the outer wilted leaves. Cut in half and set aside.

Wash the cucumber and cut into thin slices. Fill the measuring cup and reserve the rest for later. Set aside.

Now, combine zucchini, broccoli, Brussels sprouts, cucumber and ginger in a juicer and process until well juiced.

Transfer to a serving glass and add one teaspoon of olive oil before serving.

Serve immediately.

Enjoy!

Nutrition information per serving: Kcal: 160, Protein: 15.3g, Carbs: 41.5g, Fats: 1.6g

27. Avocado Asparagus Juice

Ingredients:

1 cup of fresh asparagus, trimmed

1 cup of avocado, cubed

1 small Golden Delicious apple, cored

1 whole lime, peeled

1 cup of Swiss chard, torn

1 small ginger knob, peeled

Preparation:

Wash the asparagus and trim off the woody ends. Cut into bite-sized pieces and set aside.

Peel the avocado and cut lengthwise in half. Remove the pit and cut into small chunks. Set aside.

Wash the apple and remove the core. Cut into bite-sized pieces and set aside.

Peel the lime and cut lengthwise in half. Set aside.

Rinse the Swiss chard thoroughly under cold running water and slightly drain. Torn with hands and set aside.

Peel the ginger knob and cut into small pieces. Set aside.

Now, process asparagus, avocado, apple, lime, chard, and ginger in a juicer. Transfer to a serving glass and refrigerate for 15 minutes before serving.

Enjoy!

Nutritional information per serving: Kcal: 313, Protein: 7.2g, Carbs: 46.4g, Fats: 22.5g

28. Avocado Swiss chard Juice

Ingredients:

1 cup of avocado, sliced

1 cup of Swiss chard, torn

2 medium-sized carrots

1 whole lime, peeled

1 cup of fennel, chopped

1 teaspoon of olive oil

Preparation:

Rinse the Swiss chard thoroughly under cold running water and slightly drain. Torn with hands and set aside.

Peel the avocado and cut lengthwise in half. Remove the pit and cut into thin slices. Fill the measuring cup and reserve the rest for later.

Wash and peel the carrots. Cut into small chunks and set aside.

Peel the lime and cut lengthwise in half. Set aside.

Wash the fennel bulb and trim off the wilted outer layers. Cut into small chunks and fill the measuring cup. Reserve the rest for some other juice.

Wash and peel the carrots. Cut into small chunks and set aside.

Now, combine avocado, Swiss chard, carrots, lime and fennel in a juicer and process until well juiced. Transfer to a serving glass and add one teaspoon of olive oil before serving.

Refrigerate for 15 minutes before serving.

Enjoy!

Nutritional information per serving: Kcal: 267, Protein: 6g, Carbs: 35.8g, Fats: 22.5g

29.   Avocado Zucchini Juice

Ingredients:

1 cup of avocado, chunked

1 small zucchini, chopped

1 whole lime, peeled

1 large orange, peeled

1 tsp of fresh mint, finely chopped

Preparation:

Peel the avocado and cut in half. Remove the pit and cut into chunks. Set aside.

Peel the zucchini and cut lengthwise in half. Scrape out the seeds and wash it. Cut into small pieces and set aside.

Peel the lime and cut lengthwise in half. Set aside.

Peel the orange and divide into wedges. Cut each wedge in half and set aside.

Now, combine avocado, zucchini, orange, lime, and mint in a juicer and process until juiced. Transfer to a serving glass and stir in the coconut water. Add some crushed ice and serve immediately.

Enjoy!

Nutritional information per serving: Kcal: 309, Protein: 5.8g, Carbs: 44.5g, Fats: 22.4g

30.   Avocado Fennel Juice

Ingredients:

1 cup of avocado, chunked

1 cup of fennel, chopped

1 small Granny Smith's apple, chopped

1 cup of cucumber, sliced

¼ tsp of ginger, ground

Preparation:

Peel the avocado and cut in half. Remove the pit and cut into small chunks. Fill the measuring cup and reserve the rest for later.

Wash the fennel bulb and trim off the wilted outer layers. Cut into small chunks and fill the measuring cup. Reserve the rest in the refrigerator.

Wash the apple and remove the core. Cut into bite-sized pieces and set aside.

Wash the cucumber and cut into thin slices. Fill the measuring cup and reserve the rest in the refrigerator. Set aside.

Now, combine avocado, fennel, apple, and cucumber in a juicer and process until juiced. Transfer to a serving glass and stir in the ginger.

Add some ice before serving.

Nutritional information per serving: Kcal: 286, Protein: 5g, Carbs: 40.3g, Fats: 21.9g

31.   Mustard Green Swiss Chard Juice

Ingredients:

2 cups of mustard greens, torn

2 cups of fresh spinach, torn

2 large carrots, sliced

2 cups of Swiss chard, torn

1 tsp of fresh rosemary, finely chopped

Preparation:

Wash mustard greens and spinach thoroughly under cold running water. Slightly drain and torn with hands. Set aside.

Wash the spinach thoroughly and slightly drain. Torn with hands and set aside.

Wash and peel the carrot. Cut into thin slices and set aside.

Rinse the Swiss chard thoroughly under cold running water and slightly drain. Torn with hands and set aside.

Now, combine mustard greens, spinach, carrot, Swiss chard and rosemary in a juicer and process until juiced.

Refrigerate for 15 minutes before serving.

Enjoy!

Nutritional information per serving: Kcal: 78, Protein: 7.5g, Carbs: 23.9g, Fats: 1.2g

32.   Pepper Celery Juice

Ingredients:

1 cup of fresh kale, torn

1 medium-sized celery stalk, chopped

1 cup of green peas

1 cup of fresh spinach, torn

¼ tsp of salt

Preparation:

Combine kale and spinach in a colander. Wash thoroughly under cold running water and slightly drain. Torn with hands and set aside.

Wash the celery stalk and cut into small pieces. Set aside.

Rinse the green peas using a colander. Place them in a bowl and soak in water for at least 30 minutes before using. You can also cook peas to soften. However, it's optional.

Now, combine kale, celery, peas and spinach in a juicer and process until juiced. Transfer to a serving glass and stir in the salt.

Serve immediately.

Enjoy!

Nutritional information per serving: Kcal: 166, Protein: 21g, Carbs: 41.5g, Fats: 2.6g

33.   Spinach Green Bean Juice

Ingredients:

1 cup of fresh spinach, chopped

1 cup of green beans, chopped

1 medium-sized Granny Smith's apple, cored

1 medium-sized celery stalk, cut into bite-sized pieces

1 teaspoon of olive oil

Preparation:

Wash the spinach thoroughly under cold running water. Chop into small pieces and fill the measuring cup. Reserve the rest for later.

Wash the green beans and chop into bite-sized pieces. Fill the measuring cup and reserve the rest for later.

Wash the apple and cut in half. Remove the core and cut into small chunks. Set aside.

Wash the celery and cut into bite-sized pieces. Set aside.

Now, combine spinach, green beans, apple and celery in a juicer and process until well juiced. Transfer to serving glass and add one teaspoon of olive oil before serving.

Add some ice before serving.

Enjoy!

Nutritional information per serving: Kcal: 140, Protein: 8.5g, Carbs: 37.3g, Fats: 1.4g

34. Grapefruit Blueberries Juice

Ingredients:

1 whole grapefruit, wedged

1 cup of blueberries

1 small Golden Delicious apple, cored

¼ tsp of cinnamon, ground

Preparation:

Peel the grapefruit and divide into wedges. Cut each wedge in half and set aside.

Wash the blueberries using a colander. Slightly drain and set aside.

Wash the apple and cut in half. Remove the core and cut into bite-sized pieces. Set aside.

Now, combine grapefruit, blueberries, and apple in a juicer and process until juiced. Transfer to a serving glass and stir in the cinnamon.

Add some ice before serving and enjoy!

Nutritional information per serving: Kcal: 191, Protein: 2.1g, Carbs: 54.7g, Fats: 1g

35. Avocado Cranberries Juice

Ingredients:

1 cup of avocado, cubed

1 whole lemon, peeled

1 cup of cranberries

1 cup of cucumber, sliced

1 small zucchini, chopped

1 cup of parsley, torn

Preparation:

Peel the avocado and cut into small cubes. Fill the measuring cup and reserve the rest in the refrigerator. Set aside.

Peel the lemon and cut lengthwise in half. Set aside.

Wash the cranberries and set aside.

Wash the cucumber and cut into slices. Fill the measuring cup and reserve the rest for later.

Peel the zucchini and cut into bite-sized pieces. Set aside.

Wash the parsley and torn with hands. Fill the measuring

cup and reserve the rest for later.

Now, combine avocado, cranberries, cucumber, parsley and zucchini in a juicer and process until juiced. Transfer to a serving glass and add some ice before serving.

Enjoy!

Nutritional information per serving: Kcal: 343, Protein: 8.6g, Carbs: 44.1g, Fats: 30.6g

36.   Blackberry Grapefruit Juice

Ingredients:

1 cup of blackberries

1 whole grapefruit, wedged

1 medium-sized blood orange, peeled

1 whole lemon, peeled

2 medium-sized carrots, sliced

1 oz of water

Preparation:

Wash the blackberries thoroughly under cold water and slightly drain. Set aside.

Peel the grapefruit and divide into wedges. Cut each wedge in half and set aside.

Peel the orange and divide into wedges. Cut each wedge in half and set aside.

Peel the lemon and cut lengthwise in half. Set aside.

Wash and peel the carrots. Cut into thin slices and set aside.

Now, combine blackberries, grapefruit, orange, lemon and carrots in a juicer. Process until juiced and transfer to a serving glass.

Add some ice or refrigerate for a while before serving.

Enjoy!

Nutritional information per serving: Kcal: 216, Protein: 6.9g, Carbs: 72.5g, Fats: 1.6g

37.   Granny Smith's apples Kale Juice

Ingredients:

1 cup of celery, chopped

2 small Granny Smith's apples, cored

1 cup of fresh kale, torn

1 whole lime, peeled

1 cup of broccoli, chopped

Preparation:

Wash the celery and chop into small pieces. Fill the measuring cup and set aside.

Wash the apple and cut in half. Remove the core and cut into bite-sized pieces. Set aside.

Wash the kale thoroughly under cold running water. Chop into small pieces and set aside.

Peel the lime and cut into small pieces. Set aside.

Wash the broccoli and cut into small pieces. Fill the measuring cup and reserve the rest in the refrigerator. Set aside.

Now, combine celery, apple, kale, lime and broccoli in a

juicer and process until juiced. Transfer to a serving glass and add some ice before serving.

Enjoy!

Nutritional information per serving: Kcal: 200, Protein: 7.58g, Carbs: 57.8g, Fats: 1.7g

38. Broccoli Fennel Juice

Ingredients:

1 cup of broccoli, chopped

1 cup of fennel, chopped

1 cup of Brussels sprouts, halved

1 cup of watercress, torn

1 cup of cucumber, sliced

Preparation:

Wash the broccoli and cut into small pieces. Fill the measuring cup and reserve the rest in the refrigerator. Set aside.

Wash the fennel and trim off the outer leaves. Using a sharp paring knife, cut into small pieces and fill the measuring cup. Reserve the rest for later.

Wash the Brussels sprouts and trim off the outer layers. Cut in half and set aside.

Wash the watercress thoroughly under cold running water. Slightly drain and torn with hands. Set aside.

Wash the cucumber and cut into thin slices. Fill the

measuring cup and reserve the rest for later.

Now, combine broccoli, fennel, Brussels sprouts, watercress, and cucumber in a juicer and process until juiced. Transfer to a serving glass and refrigerate for 10 minutes before serving.

Enjoy!

Nutritional information per serving: Kcal: 72, Protein: 7.7g, Carbs: 22.6g, Fats: 0.8g

39.   Beet Green Carrot Juice

Ingredients:

1 cup of beet greens, torn

2 large carrots, sliced

1 whole grapefruit, wedged

1 medium-sized green apple, cored

1 medium-sized orange, peeled

¼ tsp of ginger, ground

Preparation:

Wash the beet greens thoroughly under cold running water. Drain and torn with hands. Set aside.

Wash the carrot and cut into thin slices. Set aside.

Peel the grapefruit and divide into wedges. Cut each wedge in half and set aside.

Peel the orange and divide into wedges. Cut each wedge in half and set aside.

Wash the apple and cut lengthwise in half. Remove the core and cut into bite-sized pieces. Set aside.

Now, combine beet greens, carrot, grapefruit, apple and orange in a juicer and process until juiced.

Transfer to a serving glass and stir in the ginger.

Serve cold.

Enjoy!

Nutritional information per serving: Kcal: 293, Protein: 7g, Carbs: 90.5g, Fats: 1.4g

40.   Cucumber Collard Greens Juice

Ingredients:

1 cup of cucumber, sliced

2 cups of collard greens, chopped

1 whole lime, peeled

1 cup of Swiss chard, chopped

1 large celery stalk, chopped

1 cup of fresh parsley, torn

1 oz of water

Preparation:

Combine collard greens and Swiss chard in a large colander. Wash it under running water and slightly drain. Chop into small pieces and set aside.

Wash the cucumber and cut into thin slices. Fill the measuring cup and reserve the rest in the refrigerator.

Peel the lime and cut lengthwise in half. Set aside.

Wash the celery and cut into small pieces. Set aside.

Add parsley in a colander. Rinse well under cold running

water and torn with hands. Set aside.

Now, combine collard greens, cucumber, lime, Swiss chard, and celery in a juicer and process until juiced. Transfer to a serving glass and stir in the water and salt. Refrigerate for 10 minutes before serving.

Enjoy!

Nutritional information per serving: Kcal: 40, Protein: 3.8g, Carbs: 12.7g, Fats: 0.7g

41.   Basil Avocado Juice

Ingredients:

1 cup of fresh basil, torn

1 cup of avocado, cubed

1 cup of fresh parsley, torn

1 cup of fresh spinach, chopped

1 cup of mustard greens, torn

¼ tsp of salt

Preparation:

Combine basil, parsley, and mustard greens in a colander. Rinse well under cold running water and slightly drain. Torn with hands and set aside.

Wash the spinach leaves and chop into small pieces. Fill the measuring cup and reserve the rest for later. Set aside.

Peel the avocado and cut in half. Remove the pit and cut into small cubes. Fill the measuring cup and reserve the rest in the refrigerator. Set aside.

Now, combine basil, parsley, mustard greens, spinach and avocado in a juicer and process until well juiced. Transfer to a serving glass and stir in the reserved tomato juice and salt.

Serve cold.

Enjoy!

Nutrition information per serving: Kcal: 64, Protein: 10.9g, Carbs: 17.9g, Fats: 1.8g

42.   Blueberry Grapefruit Juice

Ingredients:

2 cups of blueberries

1 small ginger knob, peeled and chopped

1 medium-sized blood orange, peeled

1 whole grapefruit, wedged

Preparation:

Place the blueberries in a colander. Wash thoroughly under cold running water and drain. Fill the measuring cups and reserve the rest in the freezer.

Peel the ginger and cut into small pieces. Set aside.

Peel the orange and divide into wedges. Cut each wedge in half and set aside.

Peel the grapefruit and divide into wedges. Cut each wedge in half and set aside.

Now, combine blueberries, ginger, orange, and grapefruit in a juicer and process until juiced.

Transfer to a serving glass and add few ice cubes before serving.

Enjoy!

Nutritional information per serving: Kcal: 282, Protein: 5.4g, Carbs: 85.5g, Fats: 1.5g

43.   Romaine lettuce Grapefruit Juice

Ingredients:

1 whole grapefruit, wedged

1 cup of Romaine lettuce, shredded

2 medium-sized carrots, sliced

1 cup of fresh mint, chopped

1 whole lime, peeled

Preparation:

Peel the grapefruit and divide into wedges. Cut each wedge in half and set aside.

Wash the lettuce thoroughly under cold running water. Shred it and fill the measuring cup. Reserve the rest for later.

Wash and peel the carrots. Cut into thin slices and set aside.

Wash the mint and then place it in a medium bowl. Add one cup of hot water and let it soak for 10 minutes. Slightly drain and set aside.

Peel the lime and cut lengthwise in half. Set aside.

Now, combine grapefruit, lettuce, carrots, mint, and lime in a juicer and process until juiced. Transfer to a serving glass and add some crushed ice before serving.

Enjoy!

Nutritional information per serving: Kcal: 147, Protein: 4.7g, Carbs: 46.8g, Fats: 1.1g

44.   Basil Broccoli Juice

Ingredients:

2 cups of cauliflower, chopped

1 cup of fresh basil, torn

1 cup of Swiss chard, torn

1 cup of broccoli, chopped

1 cup of beet greens, torn

1 large lemon, peeled

1 medium-sized green apple, cored

Preparation:

Trim off the outer leaves of a cauliflower. Wash it and fill and cut into small pieces. Fill the measuring cup and reserve the rest in the refrigerator.

Combine basil and beet greens in a large colander. Rinse under cold running water and drain. Torn with hands and set aside.

Rinse the Swiss chard thoroughly under cold running water and slightly drain. Torn with hands and set aside.

Wash the broccoli and chop into small pieces. Set aside.

Peel the lemon and cut lengthwise in half. Set aside.

Wash the apple and cut lengthwise in half. Remove the core and cut into bite-sized pieces. Set aside.

Now, combine cauliflower, basil, broccoli, beet greens, lemon, apple and Swiss chard in a juicer. Process until well juiced and transfer to a serving glass.

Add few ice cubes and serve immediately.

Enjoy!

Nutritional information per serving: Kcal: 138, Protein: 7.4g, Carbs: 41.4g, Fats: 1.3g

45.   Brussels Sprouts Kale Juice

Ingredients:

2 cups of Brussels sprouts, halved

1 medium-sized Granny Smith's apple, cored

1 cup of fresh mint, torn

1 cup of fresh kale, torn

1 whole lime, peeled

1 cup of broccoli, chopped

1 oz of water

Preparation:

Wash the Brussels sprouts and trim off the outer leaves. Cut in half and fill the measuring cup. Reserve the rest for later.

Wash the apple and cut in half. Remove the core and cut into bite-sized pieces. Set aside.

Combine mint and kale in a large colander and rinse under cold running water. Slightly drain and torn with hands. Set aside.

Peel the lime and cut lengthwise in half. Set aside.

Wash the broccoli and chop into small pieces. Set aside.

Now, combine Brussels sprouts, apple, mint, kale, lime and broccoli in a juicer and process until juiced. Transfer to a serving glass and stir in the water.

Refrigerate for 10 minutes before serving.

Enjoy!

Nutritional information per serving: Kcal: 171, Protein: 14g, Carbs: 74.4, Fats: 2.2g

46.   Carrot Parsnip Juice

Ingredients:

2 medium-sized carrots, sliced

2 cups of parsnip, sliced

1 cup of cucumber, sliced

1 cup of watercress, torn

1 whole lemon, peeled

1 small ginger knob, peeled

1 tbsp of honey

Preparation:

Wash and peel the parsnips and carrots. Cut into thin slices and set aside.

Peel the cucumber and chop into chunks. Fill the measuring cup and reserve the rest for later.

Rinse the watercress under cold running water and slightly drain. Torn with hands and set aside.

Peel the lemon and cut lengthwise in half. Set aside.

Peel the ginger knob and cut into small pieces. Set aside.

Now, combine parsnip, carrot, cucumber, watercress, lemon, and ginger in a juicer and process until well juiced.

Transfer to a serving glass and stir in the honey.

Enjoy!

Nutritional information per serving: Kcal: 210, Protein: 6.2g, Carbs: 68.3g, Fats: 1.4g

47.   Fennel Mustard greens Juice

Ingredients:

1 cup of fennel, chopped

2 cups of mustard greens, torn

1 large leek, chopped

1 cup of fresh mint, torn

1 large green apple, cored

A handful of spinach

1 tbsp of liquid honey

Preparation:

Wash mustard greens and spinach thoroughly under cold running water. Slightly drain and torn with hands. Set aside

Wash the fennel bulb and trim off the wilted outer layers. Cut into small chunks and fill the measuring cup. Reserve the rest in the refrigerator.

Wash the leek and cut into bite-sized pieces. Set aside.

Wash the apple and cut in half. Remove the core and cut into bite-sized pieces. Set aside.

Now, combine fennel, mustard greens, mint, spinach, leek, and apple in a juicer. Process until well juiced.

Transfer to a serving glass and refrigerate for 15 minutes before serving.

Nutritional information per serving: Kcal: 180, Protein: 6.2g, Carbs: 53.7g, Fats: 1.4g

48. Kale Mustard Green Juice

Ingredients:

2 medium-sized green apples, cored

1 cup of cucumber, sliced

2 cups of fresh kale, chopped

1 cup of mustard greens, torn

1 cup of fresh spinach, torn

1 large carrot, sliced

1 tsp of fresh rosemary, finely chopped

Preparation:

Wash the apples and cut lengthwise in half. Remove the core and cut into bite-sized pieces. Set aside.

Wash the cucumber and cut into thin slices. Fill the measuring cup and reserve the rest for later. Set aside.

Wash the kale thoroughly under cold running water. Chop into small pieces and set aside.

Wash mustard greens and spinach thoroughly under cold running water. Slightly drain and torn with hands. Set aside.

Wash and peel the carrot. Cut into thin slices and set aside.

Now, combine apples, mustard greens, spinach, carrot and rosemary in a juicer and process until juiced.

Transfer to a serving glass and refrigerate for 15 minutes before serving.

Enjoy!

Nutritional information per serving: Kcal: 250, Protein: 11g, Carbs: 71.5g, Fats: 2.5g

ADDITIONAL TITLES FROM THIS AUTHOR

70 Effective Meal Recipes to Prevent and Solve Being Overweight: Burn Fat Fast by Using Proper Dieting and Smart Nutrition

By

Joe Correa CSN

48 Acne Solving Meal Recipes: The Fast and Natural Path to Fixing Your Acne Problems in Less Than 10 Days!

By

Joe Correa CSN

41 Alzheimer's Preventing Meal Recipes: Reduce or Eliminate Your Alzheimer's Condition in 30 Days or Less!

By

Joe Correa CSN

70 Effective Breast Cancer Meal Recipes: Prevent and Fight Breast Cancer with Smart Nutrition and Powerful Foods

By

Joe Correa CSN

www.ingramcontent.com/pod-product-compliance
Lightning Source LLC
Chambersburg PA
CBHW030258030426
42336CB00009B/439